EAT WELL LOSE WEIGHT COOK BOOK

A Complete Guide to Effective Intermittent Fasting for Sustainable Weight Loss.

MICHAEL JUNIOR

Copyright©2023 MICHAEL JUNIOR

TABLE OF CONTENT

INTRODUCTION

Welcome to the "Eat Well Lose Weight Cook Book: A Complete Guide to Effective Intermittent Fasting for Sustainable Weight Loss." with a society awash with dietary fads and weight-loss tactics, intermittent fasting has emerged as a compelling and long-term way to obtaining and maintaining a healthy weight.

This thorough book is intended to be a reliable companion on your road toward a better, more balanced living. Intermittent fasting is a conscious and purposeful manner of eating that taps into the body's natural cycles, providing a comprehensive approach to weight control and general well-being.

As you begin on this transforming journey, you will learn not just the science of intermittent fasting, but also practical insights, delectable recipes, and concrete recommendations to make this lifestyle more accessible and pleasurable.

We'll discuss the advantages of intermittent fasting, how to get started, and how to adjust it to your own requirements and tastes.

Our objective is to provide you with knowledge, educate you through the subtleties of intermittent fasting, and give you with the tools you need to make informed health decisions. This book is designed to inspire and assist you on your road to eating well, reducing weight, and embracing a sustainable and rewarding lifestyle, whether you are a seasoned practitioner or a newbie to the notion.

Prepare to discover the transformational power of intermittent fasting, replenish your body with nutritious meals, and begin on a road to a healthier, more vibrant self. Let's get started and learn the keys of effective intermittent fasting for long-term weight loss.

Berry and Almond Smoothie

Scenario:

Imagine starting your day with a burst of energy and a deliciously refreshing Berry and Almond Smoothie.

Packed with antioxidants, vitamins, and protein, this smoothie not only satisfies your taste buds but also provides a nutritious kick to kickstart your morning or serve as a satisfying snack.

Ingredients:

- 1 cup mixed berries (strawberries, blueberries, raspberries)
- 1 cup almond milk
- 1/2 cup Greek yogurt
- 2 tablespoons almond butter
- Ice cubes (optional)

Preparation:

Gather Ingredients: Collect all the fresh berries, almond milk, Greek yogurt, almond butter, and ice cubes.

Blend: In a blender, combine the mixed berries, almond milk, Greek yogurt, and almond butter.

Blend Until Smooth: Blend the ingredients until the mixture is smooth and creamy. Add ice cubes if you desire a colder and thicker consistency.

Adjust Consistency: If the smoothie is too thick, add more almond milk. If it's too thin, add more berries or ice cubes.

Serve: Pour the smoothie into a glass and garnish with a few whole berries for a decorative touch.

Benefits:

Rich in Antioxidants: Berries are loaded with antioxidants that help combat oxidative stress in the body, promoting overall health and well-being.

Protein Boost: Greek yogurt and almond butter add a protein boost, making this smoothie a satisfying and nourishing option, particularly for those looking to support muscle health.

Healthy Fats: Almond butter provides healthy monounsaturated fats, contributing to heart health and keeping you satiated.

Vitamins and Minerals: Berries and almond butter are rich in essential vitamins and minerals, such as vitamin C, vitamin E, and magnesium.

Low in Added Sugar: This smoothie is naturally sweetened by the berries, keeping it low in added sugars compared to store-bought alternatives.

Application:

Breakfast Boost: Kickstart your day with this smoothie for a nutritious breakfast that provides sustained energy throughout the morning.

Post-Workout Refuel: The combination of protein and carbohydrates makes this smoothie an excellent choice for replenishing energy stores after a workout.

Snack Time Delight: Combat mid-afternoon cravings by sipping on this smoothie for a tasty and satisfying snack.

On-the-Go Nutrition: Pour your smoothie into a portable cup for a convenient and healthy on-the-go option.

Roasted Brussels Sprouts with Bacon

Scenario:

Picture a cozy evening where the aroma of savory roasted Brussels sprouts and the smoky richness of bacon fill your kitchen.

This Roasted Brussels Sprouts with Bacon recipe is a delightful side dish that elevates the flavors of these cruciferous gems, making them a perfect complement to any meal.

Ingredients:

- 1 pound Brussels sprouts, trimmed and halved
- 4 slices turkey bacon, chopped
- 2 tablespoons olive oil
- Salt and pepper to taste
- Balsamic vinegar for drizzling (optional)

Preparation:

Preheat Oven: Preheat your oven to 400°F (200°C).

Prepare Brussels Sprouts: Trim the Brussels sprouts, cut them in half, and place them in a mixing bowl.

Add Bacon: In the same bowl, add chopped turkey bacon to the Brussels sprouts.

Drizzle with Olive Oil: Drizzle olive oil over the Brussels sprouts and bacon. Toss until they are evenly coated.

Season: Season with salt and pepper to taste. Toss again to ensure even seasoning.

Roast: Spread the Brussels sprouts and bacon mixture evenly on a baking sheet. Roast in the preheated oven for about 20-25 minutes or until the Brussels sprouts are golden and crispy.

Finish with Balsamic (Optional): For an extra layer of flavor, drizzle with balsamic vinegar before serving.

Serve: Transfer the roasted Brussels sprouts and bacon to a serving dish. Serve hot and enjoy!

Benefits:
High in Fiber: Brussels sprouts are rich in fiber, promoting digestive health and helping you feel full for longer periods.

Vitamins and Minerals: These little green gems are packed with vitamins C and K, as well as folate, providing essential nutrients for overall well-being.

Lean Protein: Turkey bacon adds a smoky flavor and a source of lean protein, contributing to muscle maintenance and repair.

Antioxidant Properties: Brussels sprouts contain antioxidants that help protect your cells from damage caused by free radicals.

Low in Calories: This dish is low in calories, making it a guilt-free and nutritious addition to your meal.

Application:
Holiday Side Dish: Serve this flavorful dish as a side during holiday meals or family gatherings.

Weeknight Dinner: Pair it with grilled chicken or fish for a quick and healthy weeknight dinner.

Potluck Contribution: Bring this dish to potluck dinners or picnics for a crowd-pleasing and nutritious option.

Snack or Appetizer: Enjoy roasted Brussels sprouts with bacon as a tasty and satisfying snack or appetizer.

Lemon Garlic Shrimp Skewers

Scenario:

Envision a summer barbecue or a casual dinner gathering where the tantalizing aroma of Lemon Garlic Shrimp Skewers wafts through the air.

These skewers are not only a delight for seafood enthusiasts but also a refreshing burst of flavors, perfect for a light and satisfying meal.

Ingredients:

- 1 pound large shrimp, peeled and deveined
- 3 cloves garlic, minced
- Zest of 1 lemon
- Juice of 1 lemon
- 2 tablespoons olive oil
- 1 teaspoon dried oregano
- Salt and pepper to taste
- Fresh parsley, chopped (for garnish)
- Wooden or metal skewers

Preparation:

Marinate Shrimp: In a bowl, combine the shrimp, minced garlic, lemon zest, lemon juice, olive oil, dried oregano, salt, and pepper. Toss to coat the shrimp evenly. Allow to marinate for at least 15-30 minutes.

Preheat Grill: Preheat your grill or grill pan over medium-high heat.

Skewer Shrimp: Thread the marinated shrimp onto skewers, ensuring they are evenly distributed.

Grill Shrimp: Place the shrimp skewers on the preheated grill. Grill for 2-3 minutes per side or until the shrimp turn opaque and develop a light char.

Garnish and Serve: Remove the skewers from the grill. Garnish with chopped fresh parsley and additional lemon wedges. Serve hot.

Benefits:

Lean Protein: Shrimp is a rich source of lean protein, essential for muscle health and repair.

Heart-Healthy Fats: The addition of olive oil provides heart-healthy monounsaturated fats, contributing to cardiovascular well-being.

Vitamin C Boost: The lemon juice not only adds a zesty flavor but also provides a boost of vitamin C, supporting immune function and skin health.

Quick Cooking Time: Shrimp cooks quickly, making this a time-efficient recipe, perfect for busy weeknights or last-minute gatherings.

Application:

Summer BBQ Delight: Impress your guests at summer barbecues with these flavorful shrimp skewers as a delightful appetizer or main course.

Light Dinner Option: Pair the Lemon Garlic Shrimp Skewers with a crisp salad or grilled vegetables for a light and satisfying dinner.

Appetizer for Entertaining: Serve these skewers as an elegant and tasty appetizer for dinner parties or special occasions.

Seafood Lovers' Feast: Include these skewers in a seafood-themed feast alongside other dishes like grilled fish and seafood salads.

Stuffed Bell Peppers with Quinoa and Black Beans

Scenario:

Imagine a colorful array of bell peppers, generously filled with a nutritious blend of quinoa and black beans.

These Stuffed Bell Peppers are not only a feast for the eyes but also a wholesome and flavorful dish suitable for a family dinner or a casual gathering with friends.

Ingredients:

- 4 large bell peppers, halved and seeds removed
- 1 cup cooked quinoa
- 1 can (15 oz) black beans, drained and rinsed
- 1 cup corn kernels (fresh or frozen)
- 1 cup diced tomatoes
- 1 cup shredded cheese (cheddar or Mexican blend)
- 1 teaspoon ground cumin
- 1 teaspoon chili powder
- Salt and pepper to taste
- Fresh cilantro or green onions for garnish

Preparation:

Preheat Oven: Preheat your oven to 375°F (190°C).

Prepare Bell Peppers: Cut the bell peppers in half lengthwise, removing seeds and membranes. Place them in a baking dish.

Prepare Filling: In a large bowl, combine cooked quinoa, black beans, corn, diced tomatoes, shredded cheese, ground cumin, chili powder, salt, and pepper. Mix until well combined.

Fill Peppers: Spoon the quinoa and black bean mixture into each bell pepper half, pressing down gently to pack the filling.

Bake: Cover the baking dish with foil and bake in the preheated oven for 25-30 minutes, or until the peppers are tender.

Broil (Optional): For a golden and slightly crispy top, remove the foil and broil for an additional 3-5 minutes.

Garnish and Serve: Remove from the oven, garnish with fresh cilantro or green onions, and serve hot.

Benefits:

High in Protein: The combination of quinoa and black beans provides a plant-based protein boost, supporting muscle health and keeping you satiated.

Rich in Fiber: Black beans and quinoa are excellent sources of fiber, aiding in digestion and promoting a feeling of fullness.

Vitamins and Minerals: Bell peppers contribute essential vitamins, particularly vitamin C, enhancing immune function and promoting skin health.

Low in Saturated Fat: This dish is low in saturated fat, making it a heart-healthy option for those watching their fat intake.

Vegetarian and Gluten-Free: Suitable for vegetarians and gluten-free diets, making it inclusive for various dietary preferences.

Application:

Family Dinner Favorite: Make these Stuffed Bell Peppers a regular feature for family dinners, pleasing both adults and kids alike.

Meal Prep Option: Prepare a batch for meal prep, as these stuffed peppers can be reheated for quick and nutritious lunches throughout the week.

Potluck Contribution: Bring this dish to potluck gatherings or parties, showcasing a vibrant and flavorful vegetarian option.

Pair with Sides: Serve alongside a fresh salad or avocado slices for a well-balanced and satisfying meal.

Egg and Vegetable Muffin Cups

Scenario:

Imagine a hassle-free morning where you can grab a nutritious, perfectly portioned breakfast on the go.

These Egg and Vegetable Muffin Cups are not only convenient but also customizable, providing a delicious start to your day packed with protein and veggies.

Ingredients:
- 6 large eggs
- 1/2 cup bell peppers, diced
- 1/2 cup cherry tomatoes, halved
- 1/2 cup spinach, chopped
- 1/4 cup red onion, finely chopped
- 1/4 cup feta cheese, crumbled (optional)
- Salt and pepper to taste
- Cooking spray or olive oil for greasing

Preparation:

Preheat Oven: Preheat your oven to 375°F (190°C). Grease a muffin tin with cooking spray or olive oil.

Prepare Vegetables: In a bowl, combine diced bell peppers, halved cherry tomatoes, chopped spinach, and finely chopped red onion.

Whisk Eggs: Crack the eggs into a separate bowl. Whisk them together until well combined. Season with salt and pepper.

Combine Ingredients: Add the whisked eggs to the bowl of vegetables. Mix well, ensuring an even distribution of eggs and vegetables.

Fill Muffin Cups: Pour the egg and vegetable mixture into each muffin cup, filling them about 2/3 full.

Optional Feta Topping: Sprinkle crumbled feta cheese on top of each muffin cup for added flavor (optional).

Bake: Bake in the preheated oven for 20-25 minutes or until the eggs are set and the tops are lightly golden.

Cool and Serve: Allow the muffin cups to cool for a few minutes. Use a knife to loosen the edges, and then transfer them to a plate. Serve warm.

Benefits:

Protein-Packed: Eggs are a rich source of high-quality protein, supporting muscle health and helping you feel full.

Vegetable Variety: Packed with colorful vegetables, these muffin cups provide a range of vitamins, minerals, and antioxidants for overall well-being.

Low in Carbs: Ideal for those following a low-carb or keto lifestyle, these muffin cups are satisfying without the excess carbs.

Convenient Portion Control: The muffin cup format provides convenient portion control, making it easier to manage calorie intake.

Customizable: Adapt the recipe to your taste by adding your favorite veggies or incorporating different cheese varieties.

Application:

Quick Breakfast Option: Grab one or two muffin cups for a quick and nutritious breakfast, especially on busy mornings.

Brunch Crowd-Pleaser: Serve these muffin cups at brunch gatherings for a crowd-pleasing dish that accommodates various dietary preferences.

Lunchbox Addition: Pack these muffin cups in lunchboxes for a satisfying and protein-rich midday snack.

Meal Prep Staple: Prepare a batch at the beginning of the week for easy meal prep, ensuring a healthy breakfast option is always on hand.

Tuna Salad Lettuce Wraps

Scenario:

Imagine a light and refreshing meal that combines the savory goodness of tuna salad with the crispness of fresh lettuce.

These Tuna Salad Lettuce Wraps are not only a delightful alternative to traditional sandwiches but also a nutritious option that's perfect for a quick lunch or a light dinner.

Ingredients:

- 2 cans (5 oz each) tuna in water, drained
- 1/4 cup mayonnaise
- 1 tablespoon Dijon mustard
- 1/4 cup red onion, finely diced
- 1/4 cup celery, finely diced
- 1 tablespoon fresh lemon juice
- Salt and pepper to taste
- Lettuce leaves (such as Bibb or Romaine)
- Sliced cherry tomatoes (for garnish)
- Avocado slices (optional)

Preparation:

Prepare Tuna Salad: In a bowl, combine drained tuna, mayonnaise, Dijon mustard, finely diced red onion, finely diced celery, fresh lemon juice, salt, and pepper. Mix well until all ingredients are evenly incorporated.

Chill Tuna Salad: Allow the tuna salad to chill in the refrigerator for at least 15-30 minutes to let the flavors meld.

Assemble Lettuce Wraps: Spoon the chilled tuna salad onto individual lettuce leaves, creating a generous filling.

Garnish: Top each lettuce wrap with sliced cherry tomatoes and avocado slices if desired.

Serve: Arrange the Tuna Salad Lettuce Wraps on a platter and serve immediately.

Benefits:

High-Protein: Tuna is a rich source of protein, supporting muscle health and helping to keep you feeling full and satisfied.

Low in Carbs: Lettuce wraps provide a low-carb alternative to traditional bread, making this dish suitable for those on a low-carbohydrate or keto diet.

Heart-Healthy Fats: The addition of avocado (optional) brings in heart-healthy monounsaturated fats, contributing to overall cardiovascular well-being.

Rich in Omega-3 Fatty Acids: Tuna is a good source of omega-3 fatty acids, known for their anti-inflammatory properties and benefits for heart health.

Nutrient-Packed: Celery and red onion add crunch and essential nutrients, including vitamins and antioxidants.

Application:
Lunch on the Go: Pack these wraps for a convenient and satisfying lunch, especially when you're on the go.

Light Dinner Option: Enjoy Tuna Salad Lettuce Wraps as a light and refreshing dinner option, perfect for warm evenings.

Party Appetizer: Prepare smaller wraps for a healthy and appetizing addition to parties or gatherings.

Meal Prep Staple: Make a batch of tuna salad at the beginning of the week for quick and easy assembly throughout the week.

Cucumber and Avocado Soup

Scenario:

Imagine a chilled, velvety soup that combines the cool freshness of cucumbers with the creamy texture of ripe avocados.

This Cucumber and Avocado Soup is not only a refreshing appetizer but also a nourishing dish that's perfect for hot summer days or as a light start to any meal.

Ingredients:

- 2 large cucumbers, peeled and diced
- 2 ripe avocados, peeled and pitted
- 1/2 cup Greek yogurt
- 1/4 cup fresh mint leaves
- 2 tablespoons fresh lime juice
- 1 clove garlic, minced
- 1 cup vegetable broth
- Salt and pepper to taste
- Optional garnish: cucumber slices, mint leaves, a drizzle of olive oil

Preparation:

Prepare Vegetables: Peel and dice the cucumbers. Peel and pit the avocados.

Blend Ingredients: In a blender, combine diced cucumbers, avocado, Greek yogurt, fresh mint leaves, lime juice, minced garlic, and vegetable broth. Blend until smooth and creamy.

Season: Season the soup with salt and pepper to taste. Blend again to incorporate the seasoning.

Chill: Transfer the soup to a bowl and refrigerate for at least 1-2 hours to allow it to chill and flavors to meld.

Serve: Ladle the chilled Cucumber and Avocado Soup into bowls. Garnish with cucumber slices, mint leaves, and a drizzle of olive oil if desired.

Benefits:

Hydrating: Cucumbers have high water content, making this soup a hydrating choice, especially during hot weather.

Healthy Fats: Avocados contribute heart-healthy monounsaturated fats, adding a creamy texture and providing a source of good fats.

Rich in Antioxidants: Mint leaves and avocados contain antioxidants that help combat oxidative stress and promote overall health.

Probiotics from Yogurt: Greek yogurt adds a creamy texture and provides probiotics, supporting gut health.

Vitamins and Minerals: Cucumbers and avocados are rich in vitamins and minerals, including vitamin K, vitamin C, and potassium.

Application:

Summer Appetizer: Serve this chilled soup as a refreshing appetizer at summer gatherings or barbecues.

Light Lunch Option: Enjoy a bowl of Cucumber and Avocado Soup as a light and nutritious lunch on warm days.

Starter for Dinners: Begin your dinner with this soup to stimulate the palate with its vibrant flavors.

Post-Workout Refresher: The hydrating and nutrient-packed ingredients make this soup an excellent choice for a post-workout snack.

Indulge in the cool, creamy goodness of Cucumber and Avocado Soup, a delightful and healthy addition to your culinary repertoire!

Spinach and Mushroom Stuffed Chicken Breast

Scenario:

Picture an elegant dinner with juicy chicken breasts filled with a flavorful mixture of sautéed spinach and mushrooms.

This Spinach and Mushroom Stuffed Chicken Breast is not only a feast for the eyes but also a deliciously satisfying dish that brings a touch of gourmet dining to your own kitchen.

Ingredients:

- 4 boneless, skinless chicken breasts
- 2 cups fresh spinach, chopped
- 1 cup mushrooms, finely diced
- 1/2 cup feta cheese, crumbled
- 2 cloves garlic, minced
- 1 tablespoon olive oil
- 1 teaspoon dried oregano
- Salt and pepper to taste
- Toothpicks or kitchen twine

Preparation:

Preheat Oven: Preheat your oven to 375°F (190°C).

Prepare Chicken Breasts: Lay the chicken breasts flat and carefully cut a pocket into the side of each breast, ensuring not to cut all the way through.

Sauté Spinach and Mushrooms: In a pan, heat olive oil over medium heat. Sauté chopped spinach, diced mushrooms, and minced garlic until the vegetables are soft and any excess moisture has evaporated. Season with dried oregano, salt, and pepper.

Stuff Chicken Breasts: Stuff each chicken breast pocket with the sautéed spinach and mushroom mixture. Add crumbled feta cheese to each pocket.

Secure with Toothpicks or Twine: Use toothpicks or kitchen twine to secure the openings of the stuffed chicken breasts, ensuring the filling stays inside during baking.

Season Chicken: Season the outside of each chicken breast with additional salt, pepper, and oregano.

Bake: Place the stuffed chicken breasts in a baking dish. Bake in the preheated oven for 25-30 minutes or until the chicken is cooked through and juices run clear.

Rest and Serve: Allow the stuffed chicken breasts to rest for a few minutes before removing toothpicks or twine. Slice and serve.

Benefits:

Lean Protein: Chicken breasts are a lean source of protein, supporting muscle health and aiding in weight management.

Nutrient-Packed Spinach: Spinach is rich in vitamins, minerals, and antioxidants, contributing to overall health.

Mushrooms for Immune Support: Mushrooms provide essential nutrients and may contribute to immune system support.

Feta for Calcium: Feta cheese adds a creamy texture and provides calcium for bone health.

Low Carbohydrate: This dish is low in carbohydrates, making it suitable for those following low-carb or keto diets.

Application:

Special Occasions: Impress guests with this dish as a centerpiece for special occasions or dinner parties.

Family Dinners: Make a delightful family dinner by serving Spinach and Mushroom Stuffed Chicken with your favorite sides.

Meal Prep: Prepare stuffed chicken breasts in advance for convenient and delicious meal prep throughout the week.

Date Night Dinner: Create a romantic dinner at home by serving these stuffed chicken breasts with candlelight and your favorite sides.

Indulge in the gourmet experience of Spinach and Mushroom Stuffed Chicken Breast, a dish that combines rich flavors with healthy, wholesome ingredients.

Zucchini Noodles with Pesto

Scenario:

Imagine a light and vibrant dish that replaces traditional pasta with fresh zucchini noodles, all tossed in a flavorful homemade pesto.

This Zucchini Noodles with Pesto recipe is not only a celebration of seasonal produce but also a healthy and satisfying alternative for those craving a delicious pasta experience without the carbs.

Ingredients:

For Zucchini Noodles:

- 4 medium-sized zucchini, spiralized into noodles
- Salt for seasoning

For Pesto:

- 2 cups fresh basil leaves, packed
- 1/2 cup grated Parmesan cheese
- 1/3 cup pine nuts
- 2 cloves garlic, peeled
- 1/2 cup extra-virgin olive oil
- Salt and pepper to taste
- Juice of 1 lemon (optional)

Preparation:

Prepare Zucchini Noodles: Spiralize the zucchini into noodles using a spiralizer. Sprinkle the zucchini noodles with salt and set them aside in a colander for about 15-20 minutes to allow excess moisture to drain.

Make Pesto: In a food processor, combine fresh basil, grated Parmesan cheese, pine nuts, and peeled garlic. Pulse until the ingredients are finely chopped.

Add Olive Oil: With the food processor running, slowly pour in the olive oil until the pesto reaches a smooth and creamy consistency. Season with salt and pepper to taste. Add lemon juice if desired for an extra burst of freshness.

Pat Dry Zucchini Noodles: After draining, use paper towels to pat dry the zucchini noodles, removing as much excess moisture as possible.

Toss Noodles with Pesto: In a large bowl, toss the zucchini noodles with the freshly made pesto until they are evenly coated.

Serve: Plate the Zucchini Noodles with Pesto and garnish with additional Parmesan cheese, pine nuts, or fresh basil leaves if desired.

Benefits:

Low in Calories: Zucchini noodles are a low-calorie alternative to traditional pasta, making this dish suitable for those watching their calorie intake.

Nutrient-Rich Zucchini: Zucchini is a good source of vitamins A and C, as well as potassium and dietary fiber.

Healthy Fats: The olive oil in the pesto provides heart-healthy monounsaturated fats.

Basil's Antioxidant Properties: Fresh basil contains antioxidants that help protect the body from oxidative stress.

Gluten-Free and Keto-Friendly: This dish is naturally gluten-free and fits well into a ketogenic diet.

Application:

Quick Weeknight Dinner: Whip up this dish for a quick and healthy weeknight dinner that's ready in no time.

Lunch Salad Alternative: Serve Zucchini Noodles with Pesto as a refreshing and satisfying salad alternative for lunch.

Side Dish for Grilled Proteins: Pair it with grilled chicken, shrimp, or fish for a complete and wholesome meal.

Potluck Contribution: Bring this dish to potlucks or picnics, showcasing a light and flavorful option.

Savor the freshness and flavors of summer with Zucchini Noodles with Pesto, a delightful and health-conscious twist on classic pasta dishes.

Cabbage and Turkey Sauté

Scenario:

Imagine a hearty and flavorful dish that combines the crisp texture of cabbage with seasoned ground turkey, creating a savory symphony of taste and aroma.

This Cabbage and Turkey Sauté is not only a simple and satisfying meal but also a wholesome option for those seeking a balance of protein and vegetables in their diet.

Ingredients:

- 1 pound ground turkey
- 1 small head of green cabbage, thinly sliced
- 1 cup carrots, julienned
- 1 medium onion, finely chopped
- 3 cloves garlic, minced
- 2 tablespoons soy sauce (low-sodium)
- 1 tablespoon sesame oil
- 1 teaspoon ground ginger
- Salt and pepper to taste
- Green onions for garnish (optional)
- Sesame seeds for garnish (optional)

Preparation:

Brown Turkey: In a large skillet or wok, brown the ground turkey over medium-high heat. Break it into crumbles using a spoon as it cooks.

Add Aromatics: Once the turkey is cooked, add the chopped onion, minced garlic, and ground ginger. Sauté until the onion becomes translucent and the garlic is fragrant.

Incorporate Vegetables: Add the thinly sliced cabbage and julienned carrots to the skillet. Toss and cook until the vegetables are slightly softened but still maintain a bit of crunch.

Season with Soy Sauce: Drizzle low-sodium soy sauce over the turkey and vegetables. Stir well to ensure even distribution of flavors.

Finish with Sesame Oil: Drizzle sesame oil over the sauté and toss until the ingredients are well-coated. Season with salt and pepper to taste.

Garnish and Serve: Garnish the Cabbage and Turkey Sauté with green onions and sesame seeds if desired. Serve hot.

Benefits:

Lean Protein: Ground turkey provides a lean source of protein essential for muscle health and repair.

Fiber-Rich Vegetables: Cabbage and carrots add dietary fiber, promoting digestive health and a feeling of fullness.

Low-Calorie Option: This dish is relatively low in calories, making it suitable for those watching their calorie intake.

Vitamins and Minerals: Cabbage and carrots are rich in vitamins A and C, providing essential nutrients for overall well-being.

Flavorful Seasoning: The combination of soy sauce, sesame oil, and ground ginger adds depth and flavor to the sauté.

Application:

Quick Weeknight Dinner: Prepare this sauté for a quick and nutritious weeknight dinner that's both delicious and filling.

Meal Prep Option: Make a batch and divide it into meal prep containers for convenient and healthy lunches throughout the week.

Serve Over Rice or Quinoa: Enjoy the Cabbage and Turkey Sauté over a bed of brown rice or quinoa for a wholesome and complete meal.

Asian Fusion Night: Incorporate this dish into an Asian-inspired meal alongside other favorites like stir-fried noodles or vegetable spring rolls.

Delight in the savory goodness and nutritional benefits of Cabbage and Turkey Sauté, a versatile and easy-to-make dish suitable for various occasions.

Sweet Potato and Chickpea Stew

Scenario:

Imagine a warm and comforting stew that brings together the earthy sweetness of sweet potatoes and the protein-packed goodness of chickpeas.

This Sweet Potato and Chickpea Stew is not only a hearty and flavorful meal but also a nutritious option that satisfies both the appetite and the soul.

Ingredients:

- 2 medium sweet potatoes, peeled and diced
- 1 can (15 oz) chickpeas, drained and rinsed
- 1 onion, finely chopped
- 3 cloves garlic, minced
- 1 can (14 oz) diced tomatoes
- 1 can (14 oz) coconut milk
- 1 cup vegetable broth
- 1 teaspoon ground cumin
- 1 teaspoon ground coriander
- 1 teaspoon smoked paprika
- 1/2 teaspoon turmeric
- Salt and pepper to taste

- ➢ 2 tablespoons olive oil
- ➢ Fresh cilantro for garnish (optional)

Preparation:

Sauté Aromatics: In a large pot, heat olive oil over medium heat. Sauté the chopped onion and minced garlic until softened and fragrant.

Add Spices: Add ground cumin, ground coriander, smoked paprika, and turmeric to the pot. Stir well to coat the onions and garlic with the spices.

Add Sweet Potatoes and Chickpeas: Add diced sweet potatoes and drained chickpeas to the pot. Stir to combine with the spices and aromatics.

Pour in Tomatoes, Coconut Milk, and Broth: Pour in diced tomatoes, coconut milk, and vegetable broth. Stir well, ensuring all ingredients are evenly distributed.

Simmer: Bring the stew to a gentle simmer. Cover the pot and let it cook over low heat for 20-25 minutes or until the sweet potatoes are tender.

Season and Garnish: Season the stew with salt and pepper to taste. Garnish with fresh cilantro if desired.

Serve: Ladle the Sweet Potato and Chickpea Stew into bowls and serve hot. It pairs well with rice, quinoa, or crusty bread.

Benefits:

Rich in Fiber: Sweet potatoes and chickpeas are excellent sources of dietary fiber, supporting digestive health and providing a feeling of fullness.

Protein-Packed Chickpeas: Chickpeas are a plant-based protein source, contributing to muscle health and satiety.

Vitamins and Minerals: Sweet potatoes offer a variety of vitamins, including A and C, as well as minerals like potassium.

Anti-Inflammatory Properties: Turmeric, a spice in this stew, contains curcumin, known for its anti-inflammatory properties.

Heart-Healthy Coconut Milk: Coconut milk adds a rich and creamy texture while providing heart-healthy fats.

Application:

Meatless Monday Dinner: Enjoy this stew as a hearty and satisfying meatless option for your Meatless Monday meals.

Weeknight Comfort Food: Whip up this stew for a quick and comforting dinner on busy weeknights.

Meal Prep for Lunch: Divide the stew into meal prep containers for nutritious and convenient lunches throughout the week.

Family Gatherings: Serve this flavorful stew at family gatherings or potluck dinners for a dish that caters to various dietary preferences.

Experience the warmth and nourishment of Sweet Potato and Chickpea Stew, a comforting bowl that combines flavors, textures, and health benefits in every spoonful.

Baked Cod with Lemon and Herbs

Scenario:

Picture a light and flavorful dish where the delicate taste of cod is enhanced by zesty lemon and aromatic herbs.

This Baked Cod with Lemon and Herbs is not only a simple and elegant entrée but also a healthy choice for those seeking a delicious and nutritious seafood option.

Ingredients:

- 4 cod fillets (about 6 oz each)
- 2 tablespoons olive oil
- Zest of 1 lemon
- Juice of 1 lemon
- 2 cloves garlic, minced
- 1 tablespoon fresh parsley, chopped
- 1 tablespoon fresh dill, chopped
- Salt and pepper to taste
- Lemon slices for garnish

Preparation:

Preheat Oven: Preheat your oven to 375°F (190°C).

Prepare Cod Fillets: Pat dry the cod fillets with paper towels. Place them on a baking dish lined with parchment paper or lightly greased.

Prepare Marinade: In a small bowl, whisk together olive oil, lemon zest, lemon juice, minced garlic, chopped parsley, chopped dill, salt, and pepper.

Marinate Cod: Brush the cod fillets with the lemon and herb marinade, ensuring they are evenly coated. Reserve some of the marinade for later use.

Bake: Bake the cod fillets in the preheated oven for 12-15 minutes or until the fish is opaque and flakes easily with a fork.

Broil (Optional): For a golden finish, broil the cod fillets for an additional 2-3 minutes, watching carefully to prevent burning.

Garnish and Serve: Remove the baked cod from the oven, garnish with lemon slices and additional fresh herbs. Drizzle the reserved marinade over the top before serving.

Benefits:

Lean Protein: Cod is a low-fat source of protein, contributing to muscle health and providing essential amino acids.

Rich in Omega-3 Fatty Acids: Cod is a good source of omega-3 fatty acids, known for their cardiovascular benefits and anti-inflammatory properties.

Vitamin C Boost: Lemon adds a burst of vitamin C to the dish, promoting immune health and enhancing iron absorption.

Herbs for Flavor and Antioxidants: Fresh parsley and dill not only add flavor but also contribute antioxidants and other beneficial compounds.

Heart-Healthy Olive Oil: The use of olive oil provides heart-healthy monounsaturated fats, supporting cardiovascular well-being.

Application:

Light Weeknight Dinner: Baked Cod with Lemon and Herbs is perfect for a quick and light weeknight dinner that's ready in under 30 minutes.

Elegant Dinner Parties: Impress guests with this elegant yet simple dish as the centerpiece for dinner parties or special occasions.

Healthy Holiday Option: Incorporate this baked cod into your holiday menu for a lighter and healthier alternative to heavier dishes.

Meal Prep for Lunch: Prepare extra servings for meal prep, allowing you to enjoy a healthy and delicious lunch throughout the week.

Delight in the exquisite flavors of Baked Cod with Lemon and Herbs, a dish that showcases the natural goodness of fresh fish complemented by the brightness of citrus and aromatic herbs.

Vegetarian Chili

Scenario:

Imagine a hearty bowl filled with a medley of colorful vegetables, beans, and savory spices— a dish that warms you from the inside out.

This Vegetarian Chili is not only a flavorful and satisfying comfort food but also a nutritious option that caters to various dietary preferences.

Ingredients:

- 1 tablespoon olive oil
- 1 large onion, diced
- 3 cloves garlic, minced
- 1 bell pepper, diced (choose your favorite color)
- 1 zucchini, diced
- 1 carrot, diced
- 1 can (15 oz) black beans, drained and rinsed
- 1 can (15 oz) kidney beans, drained and rinsed
- 1 can (15 oz) diced tomatoes
- 1 cup corn kernels (fresh, frozen, or canned)
- 2 tablespoons tomato paste
- 1 tablespoon chili powder
- 1 teaspoon ground cumin

- ➢ 1 teaspoon smoked paprika
- ➢ 1/2 teaspoon dried oregano
- ➢ Salt and pepper to taste
- ➢ 4 cups vegetable broth
- ➢ Fresh cilantro, chopped (for garnish)
- ➢ Avocado slices (for garnish)
- ➢ Shredded cheese (optional, for topping)
- ➢ Greek yogurt or sour cream (optional, for topping)

Preparation:

Sauté Aromatics: In a large pot, heat olive oil over medium heat. Sauté diced onion until softened, then add minced garlic and sauté for an additional 1-2 minutes until fragrant.

Add Vegetables: Add diced bell pepper, zucchini, and carrot to the pot. Sauté until the vegetables are slightly tender.

Combine Beans and Tomatoes: Stir in black beans, kidney beans, diced tomatoes, and corn. Mix well.

Season the Chili: Add tomato paste, chili powder, ground cumin, smoked paprika, dried oregano, salt, and pepper. Mix thoroughly to evenly distribute the spices.

Pour in Vegetable Broth: Pour vegetable broth into the pot and bring the mixture to a boil. Reduce the heat to low, cover, and let it simmer for at least 20-30 minutes, allowing the flavors to meld.

Adjust Seasoning: Taste the chili and adjust the seasoning as needed. If you prefer a spicier chili, you can add more chili powder or a dash of hot sauce.

Serve: Ladle the Vegetarian Chili into bowls. Garnish with chopped fresh cilantro, avocado slices, and, if desired, shredded cheese or a dollop of Greek yogurt or sour cream.

Benefits:

Plant-Based Protein: Beans and vegetables provide plant-based protein, making this chili a satisfying meatless option.

Fiber-Rich: Loaded with fiber from beans and vegetables, this chili supports digestive health and helps keep you full.

Rich in Vitamins and Minerals: Bell peppers, zucchini, and carrots add a variety of vitamins and minerals, contributing to overall well-being.

Low in Saturated Fat: Being plant-based, this chili is naturally low in saturated fat, making it a heart-healthy choice.

Versatile: Easily customizable, you can add other vegetables or spices to suit your taste preferences.

Application:
Game Day Favorite: Serve this Vegetarian Chili during game days or gatherings as a hearty and crowd-pleasing dish.

Meatless Monday Dinner: Make this chili a staple for Meatless Mondays, providing a flavorful and nutritious alternative to meat-based meals.

Meal Prep Option: Prepare a large batch for meal prep, allowing you to enjoy convenient and nutritious lunches throughout the week.

Family Dinner Delight: Enjoy this chili as a wholesome family dinner, paired with your favorite toppings and sides.

Savor the warmth and goodness of Vegetarian Chili, a comforting bowl that's not only delicious but also packed with nutritious ingredients.

Greek Yogurt Parfait

Scenario:

Picture a delightful and wholesome treat that combines the creamy goodness of Greek yogurt with layers of vibrant fruits, crunchy granola, and a drizzle of honey.

This Greek Yogurt Parfait is not only a visually appealing dessert but also a nutritious and satisfying option for breakfast or snack time.

Ingredients:

- 2 cups Greek yogurt (plain or flavored)
- 1 cup granola (choose your favorite flavor)
- 1 cup mixed berries (strawberries, blueberries, raspberries)
- 1 banana, sliced
- 1/4 cup nuts (almonds, walnuts, or your choice), chopped
- Honey for drizzling
- Fresh mint leaves for garnish (optional)

Preparation:

Choose Serving Glasses or Bowls: Select individual glasses or bowls for assembling the parfaits.

Layer Greek Yogurt: Begin by adding a layer of Greek yogurt at the bottom of each glass or bowl.

Add Granola Layer: Sprinkle a layer of granola on top of the Greek yogurt. Ensure an even distribution for a balanced bite.

Layer with Mixed Berries: Add a generous layer of mixed berries, distributing them evenly to cover the granola.

Add Banana Slices: Place slices of banana on top of the berry layer. This adds a natural sweetness and a creamy texture.

Repeat Layers: Repeat the layers until you reach the top of the glass or bowl. Finish with a dollop of Greek yogurt on the top layer.

Garnish: Sprinkle chopped nuts over the final layer and drizzle honey on top. Garnish with fresh mint leaves if desired.

Serve: Serve the Greek Yogurt Parfait immediately for a delightful and refreshing treat.

Benefits:

Protein-Rich Greek Yogurt: Greek yogurt is a high-protein dairy product that supports muscle health and helps keep you feeling full.

Fiber from Granola and Fruits: Granola and mixed berries contribute dietary fiber, aiding in digestion and promoting satiety.

Antioxidant-Rich Berries: Mixed berries, such as strawberries, blueberries, and raspberries, are rich in antioxidants that support overall health.

Potassium from Bananas: Bananas provide potassium, an essential mineral for heart health and proper muscle function.

Healthy Fats from Nuts: Chopped nuts add a satisfying crunch and provide healthy fats, contributing to overall well-being.

Application:

Quick Breakfast Option: Enjoy a Greek Yogurt Parfait as a quick and nutritious breakfast, especially on busy mornings.

Afternoon Snack: Satisfy your sweet cravings with a healthy Greek Yogurt Parfait as an afternoon snack.

Dessert Alternative: Serve these parfaits as a wholesome dessert option for family dinners or gatherings.

Brunch Spread: Include Greek Yogurt Parfaits in your brunch spread for a colorful and refreshing addition.

Create a visual feast with layers of flavor and nutrition in every spoonful of Greek Yogurt Parfait, a versatile and delightful treat suitable for various occasions.

Cauliflower Fried Rice

Scenario:

Imagine a flavorful and satisfying dish that captures the essence of fried rice but with a healthy twist.

This Cauliflower Fried Rice is not only a delicious alternative for those seeking a low-carb option but also a versatile and nutritious meal that can be customized to suit your taste preferences.

Ingredients:

- 1 medium-sized cauliflower head, grated or processed into rice-sized grains
- 2 tablespoons vegetable oil
- 1 onion, finely chopped
- 2 cloves garlic, minced
- 1 cup carrots, finely diced
- 1 cup peas (fresh or frozen)
- 2 eggs, lightly beaten
- 3 tablespoons soy sauce (low-sodium)
- 1 tablespoon sesame oil
- 1 teaspoon ginger, grated
- 4 green onions, chopped
- Salt and pepper to taste
- Optional: Protein of choice (chicken, shrimp, tofu)
- Optional: Chopped cilantro or parsley for garnish

Preparation:

Prepare Cauliflower Rice: Grate or process the cauliflower into rice-sized grains using a food processor. Set aside.

Sauté Aromatics: In a large skillet or wok, heat vegetable oil over medium heat. Add chopped onions and minced garlic. Sauté until the onions become translucent.

Add Vegetables: Add finely diced carrots and peas to the skillet. Cook for 3-4 minutes until the vegetables are tender but still slightly crisp.

Push Vegetables to One Side: Push the vegetable mixture to one side of the skillet, creating space for the eggs.

Cook Eggs: Pour the beaten eggs into the cleared side of the skillet. Allow them to set for a moment, then scramble them until cooked through.

Combine with Vegetables: Mix the cooked eggs with the vegetable mixture in the skillet.

Add Cauliflower Rice: Add the cauliflower rice to the skillet. Stir well to combine with the vegetables and eggs.

Season with Soy Sauce and Sesame Oil: Drizzle soy sauce and sesame oil over the cauliflower rice. Add grated ginger. Mix thoroughly to coat all ingredients evenly.

Adjust Seasoning: Season with salt and pepper to taste. Adjust the soy sauce or sesame oil if needed.

Add Protein (Optional): If desired, add cooked chicken, shrimp, or tofu to the cauliflower rice. Toss until well combined and heated through.

Finish with Green Onions: Stir in chopped green onions and cook for an additional 1-2 minutes.

Garnish and Serve: Garnish the Cauliflower Fried Rice with chopped cilantro or parsley if desired. Serve hot.

Benefits:

Low-Carb Alternative: Cauliflower rice is a low-carb alternative to traditional rice, making this dish suitable for low-carb and keto diets.

Rich in Fiber: Cauliflower provides dietary fiber, aiding in digestion and promoting a feeling of fullness.

Versatile and Customizable: You can customize this dish by adding your favorite protein or additional vegetables to suit your taste preferences.

Reduced Sodium Option: Using low-sodium soy sauce allows you to control the sodium content of the dish.

Packed with Vegetables: The inclusion of carrots, peas, and green onions adds a variety of vitamins, minerals, and antioxidants.

Application:
Quick Weeknight Dinner: Cauliflower Fried Rice is a quick and easy weeknight dinner that comes together in under 30 minutes.

Meal Prep Option: Prepare a batch for meal prep, ensuring convenient and healthy lunches throughout the week.

Side Dish for Asian-Inspired Meals: Serve Cauliflower Fried Rice as a delicious side dish for your favorite Asian-inspired meals.

Vegetarian Option: Enjoy this dish as a satisfying vegetarian meal or alongside other vegetarian dishes.

Mushroom and Spinach Omelette

Scenario:

Envision a nutritious and flavorful breakfast that combines earthy mushrooms, vibrant spinach, and fluffy eggs.

This Mushroom and Spinach Omelette is not only a quick and satisfying morning option but also a versatile dish that caters to various tastes and dietary preferences.

Ingredients:

- 3 large eggs
- 1 cup fresh spinach, chopped
- 1/2 cup mushrooms, sliced
- 1/4 cup onion, finely chopped
- 1 clove garlic, minced
- 1 tablespoon butter or olive oil
- Salt and pepper to taste
- 1/4 cup shredded cheese (cheddar, feta, or your preference)
- Fresh herbs (parsley or chives) for garnish (optional)
- Salsa or hot sauce for serving (optional)

Preparation:

Sauté Mushrooms and Onions: In a non-stick skillet, heat butter or olive oil over medium heat. Sauté sliced mushrooms and chopped onions until they are softened and lightly browned.

Add Garlic and Spinach: Add minced garlic to the skillet and stir until fragrant. Add chopped spinach and cook until wilted. Season with salt and pepper to taste.

Whisk Eggs: In a bowl, whisk the eggs until well beaten. Season with a pinch of salt.

Pour Eggs into Skillet: Pour the beaten eggs over the sautéed mushrooms, onions, and spinach. Allow the eggs to set around the edges.

Gently Lift and Tilt: Gently lift the edges of the omelette with a spatula, tilting the skillet to let the uncooked eggs flow to the edges.

Add Cheese: Sprinkle shredded cheese over one half of the omelette.

Fold and Serve: Once the eggs are mostly set but still slightly runny on top, carefully fold the omelette in half with the spatula. Continue cooking until the eggs are fully set and the cheese is melted.

Garnish and Serve: Slide the Mushroom and Spinach Omelette onto a plate. Garnish with fresh herbs if desired. Serve hot with salsa or hot sauce on the side if you like a bit of heat.

Benefits:

Protein-Rich: Eggs provide high-quality protein, essential for muscle health and satiety.

Iron and Fiber from Spinach: Spinach is rich in iron and dietary fiber, supporting energy levels and digestive health.

Antioxidant-Rich Mushrooms: Mushrooms contribute antioxidants and various nutrients that support overall well-being.

Healthy Fats: Olive oil or butter provides healthy fats that aid in nutrient absorption and satiety.

Versatile and Customizable: This omelette is easily customizable with additional vegetables, herbs, or different types of cheese.

Application:

Quick Breakfast Option: Prepare this Mushroom and Spinach Omelette for a quick and nutritious breakfast to start your day.

Brunch Delight: Serve this omelette as part of a delicious brunch spread, complemented by fresh fruit and whole-grain toast.

Light Lunch or Dinner: Enjoy the omelette as a light and satisfying lunch or dinner option.

Meal Prep for Busy Mornings: Make a batch of sautéed mushrooms and onions in advance for quicker omelette preparation on busy mornings.

Experience the delightful combination of mushrooms, spinach, and eggs in this Mushroom and Spinach Omelette—a wholesome and flavorful way to kickstart your day.

Turkey and Vegetable Stir-Fry

Scenario:

Visualize a colorful and savory stir-fry that brings together lean turkey, crisp vegetables, and a deliciously seasoned sauce.

This Turkey and Vegetable Stir-Fry is not only a quick and wholesome meal option but also a versatile dish that allows you to enjoy the vibrant flavors of fresh ingredients in every bite.

Ingredients:

- 1 pound ground turkey
- 2 tablespoons soy sauce (low-sodium)
- 1 tablespoon oyster sauce
- 1 tablespoon hoisin sauce
- 1 tablespoon sesame oil
- 1 tablespoon vegetable oil
- 3 cloves garlic, minced
- 1 tablespoon ginger, grated
- 1 onion, thinly sliced
- 1 bell pepper, thinly sliced (use your preferred color)
- 1 zucchini, thinly sliced
- 1 carrot, julienned
- 1 cup broccoli florets
- 1 cup snap peas, ends trimmed
- Cooked rice or noodles for serving

> ➢ Sesame seeds and chopped green onions for garnish (optional)

Preparation:

Prepare Sauce: In a small bowl, whisk together soy sauce, oyster sauce, hoisin sauce, and sesame oil. Set aside.

Cook Ground Turkey: In a large wok or skillet, heat vegetable oil over medium-high heat. Add ground turkey and cook, breaking it into crumbles, until browned and cooked through.

Add Aromatics: Push the cooked turkey to one side of the wok. Add minced garlic and grated ginger to the cleared side. Sauté until fragrant.

Add Vegetables: Add thinly sliced onion, bell pepper, zucchini, julienned carrot, broccoli florets, and snap peas to the wok. Stir-fry for 3-5 minutes or until the vegetables are tender-crisp.

Combine and Stir: Combine the cooked turkey with the sautéed vegetables in the wok. Stir to evenly distribute the ingredients.

Pour in Sauce: Pour the prepared sauce over the turkey and vegetables. Stir well, ensuring everything is coated in the flavorful sauce. Cook for an additional 2-3 minutes.

Check Seasoning: Taste and adjust the seasoning if needed. You can add more soy sauce or other sauces according to your taste preferences.

Serve: Serve the Turkey and Vegetable Stir-Fry over cooked rice or noodles. Garnish with sesame seeds and chopped green onions if desired.

Benefits:

Lean Protein: Ground turkey serves as a lean source of protein, essential for muscle health and repair.

Colorful Vegetables: A variety of vegetables provide essential vitamins, minerals, and antioxidants, contributing to overall well-being.

Healthy Fats: Sesame oil adds a rich and nutty flavor while providing heart-healthy fats.

Low in Sodium Option: Using low-sodium soy sauce allows you to control the sodium content of the dish.

Customizable: You can customize the stir-fry by adding your favorite vegetables or adjusting the level of spiciness.

Application:

Quick Weeknight Dinner: Enjoy this Turkey and Vegetable Stir-Fry as a quick and wholesome dinner option on busy weeknights.

Meal Prep for Lunch: Prepare a batch for meal prep, allowing you to enjoy delicious and nutritious lunches throughout the week.

Protein-Packed Stir-Fry: Incorporate this stir-fry into your fitness routine as a protein-packed and satisfying post-workout meal.

Family-Friendly Dish: Serve this stir-fry as a family-friendly dinner, appealing to both adults and kids.

Savor the delightful combination of turkey, vibrant vegetables, and savory sauce in this Turkey and Vegetable Stir-Fry—a versatile and nutritious dish that brings joy to your taste buds.

Salmon and Asparagus Foil Pack

Scenario:

Imagine a hassle-free and flavorful dish where succulent salmon fillets and crisp asparagus are perfectly seasoned and cooked to perfection, all within a convenient foil pack.

This Salmon and Asparagus Foil Pack is not only a simple and delicious dinner option but also a no-fuss way to enjoy the health benefits of fresh fish and vegetables.

Ingredients:

- 4 salmon fillets
- 1 bunch fresh asparagus, trimmed
- 3 tablespoons olive oil
- 3 cloves garlic, minced
- 1 lemon, sliced
- 2 tablespoons fresh dill, chopped
- Salt and pepper to taste
- Optional: Red pepper flakes for a hint of spice
- Optional: Sliced cherry tomatoes for added freshness

Preparation:

Preheat Oven: Preheat your oven to 400°F (200°C).

Prepare Foil Packets: Cut four large squares of aluminum foil. Place a salmon fillet in the center of each foil square.

Season Salmon: Drizzle each salmon fillet with olive oil. Sprinkle minced garlic, chopped dill, salt, and pepper over the salmon. Add a pinch of red pepper flakes if desired.

Arrange Asparagus: Place a handful of trimmed asparagus next to each salmon fillet. Ensure that the asparagus is evenly distributed.

Top with Lemon Slices: Lay lemon slices over the salmon fillets and asparagus. The lemon not only adds flavor but also keeps the salmon moist during cooking.

Seal Foil Packets: Fold the foil over the salmon and asparagus, creating a sealed packet. Ensure that the packets are well-sealed to trap in the flavors and juices.

Bake: Place the foil packets on a baking sheet and bake in the preheated oven for 15-20 minutes or until the salmon is cooked through and flakes easily with a fork.

Optional Tomato Garnish: If desired, open the foil packets during the last few minutes of cooking and add sliced cherry tomatoes for a burst of freshness.

Serve: Carefully open the foil packets, transfer the salmon, asparagus, and lemon slices to plates, and spoon any accumulated juices over the top.

Benefits:

Omega-3 Fatty Acids: Salmon is rich in omega-3 fatty acids, known for their heart-healthy benefits and anti-inflammatory properties.

Lean Protein: Salmon provides a lean source of protein, essential for muscle health and overall well-being.

Vitamins and Minerals: Asparagus contributes vitamins A, C, and K, as well as folate and potassium, enhancing the nutritional profile of the dish.

Antioxidants: Garlic, lemon, and fresh dill add antioxidants, supporting immune health and providing additional flavor.

Low in Carbs: This dish is naturally low in carbohydrates, making it suitable for various dietary preferences.

Application:

Effortless Weeknight Dinner: The Salmon and Asparagus Foil Pack is perfect for a quick and effortless weeknight dinner that requires minimal cleanup.

Outdoor Grilling: Take this foil pack recipe outdoors and cook it on the grill for a delightful summer meal with a smoky flavor.

Healthy Meal Prep: Prepare multiple foil packs and store them in the refrigerator for easy and healthy meal prep throughout the week.

Dinner Party Delight: Impress guests with an elegant and flavorful presentation by serving individual foil packs at your next dinner party.

Indulge in the simplicity and freshness of the Salmon and Asparagus Foil Pack—a delightful and wholesome dish that allows the natural flavors of the ingredients to shine.

Quinoa and Black Bean Bowl:

Scenario:

Visualize a vibrant and nourishing bowl where fluffy quinoa, protein-packed black beans, and an array of colorful vegetables come together to create a wholesome and satisfying meal.

This Quinoa and Black Bean Bowl is not only a delicious option for those seeking plant-based goodness but also a versatile dish that can be customized to suit your taste preferences.

Ingredients:

- 1 cup quinoa, rinsed
- 2 cups water or vegetable broth
- 1 can (15 oz) black beans, drained and rinsed
- 1 cup cherry tomatoes, halved
- 1 bell pepper (any color), diced
- 1 avocado, sliced
- 1 cup corn kernels (fresh, frozen, or canned)
- 1/4 cup red onion, finely chopped
- Fresh cilantro, chopped, for garnish
- Lime wedges for serving

For the Lime-Cilantro Dressing:

- 3 tablespoons olive oil
- Juice of 2 limes

- ➤ 1 clove garlic, minced
- ➤ 1 tablespoon fresh cilantro, chopped
- ➤ Salt and pepper to taste

Preparation:

Cook Quinoa: In a medium saucepan, combine quinoa and water or vegetable broth. Bring to a boil, then reduce heat to low, cover, and simmer for 15-20 minutes, or until the quinoa is cooked and the liquid is absorbed. Fluff the quinoa with a fork.

Prepare Lime-Cilantro Dressing: In a small bowl, whisk together olive oil, lime juice, minced garlic, chopped cilantro, salt, and pepper. Set aside.

Assemble Bowl: In individual serving bowls, layer the cooked quinoa, black beans, cherry tomatoes, diced bell pepper, avocado slices, corn kernels, and chopped red onion.

Drizzle with Dressing: Drizzle the Lime-Cilantro Dressing over the quinoa and black bean bowl.

Garnish and Serve: Garnish the bowl with fresh cilantro and serve with lime wedges on the side.

Benefits:

Complete Protein: Quinoa and black beans together form a complete protein, providing all essential amino acids for vegetarians and vegans.

Fiber-Rich: Black beans and quinoa are rich in dietary fiber, promoting digestive health and aiding in satiety.

Abundance of Vitamins and Minerals: The variety of vegetables in the bowl contribute vitamins, such as C and A, as well as minerals like potassium.

Healthy Fats: Avocado adds heart-healthy monounsaturated fats, enhancing the overall nutritional profile.

Customizable and Adaptable: This bowl is easily adaptable to personal preferences—you can add or substitute ingredients based on what you have on hand.

Application:

Meatless Monday Dinner: Enjoy this Quinoa and Black Bean Bowl as a satisfying and meatless option for your Meatless Monday meals.

Work Lunch or Dinner: Prepare a batch of these bowls for convenient and nutritious work lunches or dinners.

Picnic or Outdoor Gathering: Pack the components separately and assemble the bowls during a picnic or outdoor gathering for a fresh and wholesome meal.

Family-Friendly Meal: Customize the bowl with various toppings and allow family members to create their own personalized versions.

Experience the delightful combination of flavors, textures, and health benefits in every bite of this Quinoa and Black Bean Bowl—a versatile and nutritious dish that brings together the goodness of plant-based ingredients.

Grilled Chicken Salad with Lemon Vinaigrette

Scenario:

Imagine a light and refreshing salad where perfectly grilled chicken meets a colorful medley of fresh vegetables, all tossed in a zesty lemon vinaigrette.

This Grilled Chicken Salad is not only a delightful combination of flavors and textures but also a nourishing and satisfying meal that's perfect for any occasion.

Ingredients:

For the Grilled Chicken:

- 4 boneless, skinless chicken breasts
- 2 tablespoons olive oil
- 1 teaspoon dried oregano
- 1 teaspoon garlic powder
- Salt and pepper to taste

For the Salad:

- Mixed salad greens (lettuce, spinach, arugula, etc.)
- Cherry tomatoes, halved
- Cucumber, sliced
- Red bell pepper, thinly sliced
- Red onion, thinly sliced
- Avocado, sliced

> ➤ Feta cheese, crumbled
> ➤ Kalamata olives, pitted
> ➤ Fresh parsley, chopped (for garnish)

For the Lemon Vinaigrette:
> ➤ 1/4 cup olive oil
> ➤ Juice of 1 lemon
> ➤ 1 teaspoon Dijon mustard
> ➤ 1 clove garlic, minced
> ➤ Salt and pepper to taste

Preparation:

Marinate Chicken: In a bowl, mix olive oil, dried oregano, garlic powder, salt, and pepper. Coat the chicken breasts with this marinade and let them marinate for at least 30 minutes.

Preheat Grill: Preheat the grill to medium-high heat.

Grill Chicken: Grill the marinated chicken breasts for 6-8 minutes per side or until fully cooked, with grill marks and an internal temperature of 165°F (74°C). Allow the chicken to rest for a few minutes before slicing.

Prepare Salad Greens: In a large salad bowl, combine mixed greens, halved cherry tomatoes, cucumber slices, red bell pepper slices, red onion slices, avocado slices, crumbled feta cheese, and Kalamata olives.

Slice Grilled Chicken: Slice the grilled chicken breasts into thin strips.

Assemble Salad: Arrange the sliced grilled chicken over the salad greens and vegetables.

Prepare Lemon Vinaigrette: In a small bowl, whisk together olive oil, lemon juice, Dijon mustard, minced garlic, salt, and pepper to create the vinaigrette.

Dress Salad: Drizzle the lemon vinaigrette over the salad, tossing gently to coat all ingredients evenly.

Garnish and Serve: Garnish the Grilled Chicken Salad with chopped fresh parsley. Serve immediately.

Benefits:

Lean Protein: Grilled chicken serves as a lean source of protein, crucial for muscle health and satiety.

Abundance of Vegetables: The colorful array of vegetables adds vitamins, minerals, and antioxidants to support overall well-being.

Healthy Fats: Avocado provides healthy monounsaturated fats, contributing to heart health.

Feta for Calcium: Feta cheese adds a touch of calcium to support bone health.

Light and Refreshing: The lemon vinaigrette not only enhances the flavor but also provides a refreshing and light dressing.

Application:

Summer Dinner Delight: Enjoy this Grilled Chicken Salad as a light and flavorful dinner option, perfect for warm summer evenings.

Lunchbox Favorite: Pack this salad in a lunchbox for a satisfying and nutritious lunch at work or school.

Impressive Entertaining Dish: Serve this salad at gatherings or dinner parties for a visually appealing and impressive dish.

Post-Workout Meal: With its protein content, this salad is an excellent choice for a post-workout meal to aid in muscle recovery.

CONCLUSION

As we come to the end of "Eat Well Lose Weight Cook Book: A Complete Guide to Effective Intermittent Fasting for Sustainable Weight Loss," we hope that this book has been a great resource on your quest to a better and more balanced life.

Intermittent fasting is more than just a quick fix; it's a way of life that promotes thoughtful and purposeful eating, supporting a long-term approach to weight management. We've refuted fallacies about intermittent fasting and offered practical advice for effective adoption throughout this book.

Remember that health and happiness are lifelong goals, and the decisions we make today set the groundwork for a prosperous tomorrow. Embracing intermittent fasting is about fueling your body with the proper meals at the right times, encouraging both physical and mental health.

As you go, personalize your intermittent fasting journey to your own requirements and tastes. Experiment with different fasting regimens, enjoy the tasty and healthy foods, and pay attention to your body's messages. Intermittent fasting is a tool, and it works best when used with understanding, attention, and consistency.

Celebrate your victories, learn from your mistakes, and be kind to yourself along the journey. Sustainable weight reduction is a comprehensive activity that includes more than just the scale—it includes the everyday decisions we make, the food we provide our bodies, and the mentality we create toward our well-being.

Thank you for entrusting us with your transformational journey. May this handbook provide you with the knowledge and motivation you need to make educated health decisions. Here's to a future of healthy eating, long-term weight loss, and a life well-lived.

I wish you continued success on your journey to better health and fitness.